S

IN **one**

hour

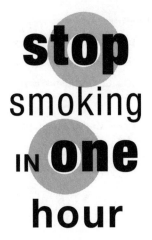

stop
smoking
IN one
hour

play the cd ... just
once ... and never
smoke again!

with

susan hepburn

Thorsons

Thorsons
An Imprint of HarperCollins*Publishers*
77–85 Fulham Palace Road,
Hammersmith, London W6 8JB

The Thorsons website address is: www.thorsons.com

Published by Thorsons 2000

10 9 8 7 6 5 4 3 2 1

© Susan Hepburn 2000

Susan Hepburn asserts the moral right to
be identified as the author of this work

A catalogue record for this book
is available from the British Library

ISBN 0 00 710406 5

Printed and bound in Great Britain by
Martins the Printers Ltd, Berwick upon Tweed

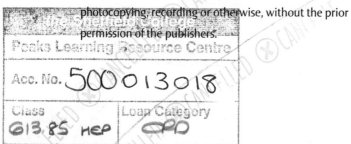

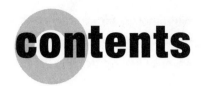

contents

introduction

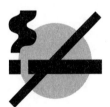 Thank you for purchasing my book and CD, please enjoy reading and, more importantly, **enjoy being a non-smoker...**

Is this Treatment a Miracle Cure?

I do not consider my treatment to be a miracle cure, although when you experience how easily you have become a non-smoker you may be tempted to consider that a miracle has happened.

Indeed you can become a non-smoker within one hour, *the time it takes to read Part One of this book and listen to my CD once only.*

You will be surprised to discover that there are no side-effects and there will be no cravings. The two main problems associated with becoming a non-smoker – irritability and nibbling between meals –

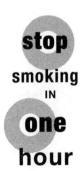

stop smoking IN **one hour**

To succeed you
need commitment and
determination.

Willpower is not required.

If you had the willpower
you would not need
my help.

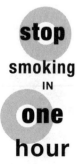

stop
smoking
IN
one
hour

are dealt with during the treatment and therefore you need not concern yourself with these issues.

Also, willpower is not required, because I believe that if you had the willpower to become a non-smoker you would not be enlisting my help. However, you do have to play your part. I cannot do it for you.

The fundamental requirements for this treatment to be successful are simply:

 your desire to be a non-smoker *for yourself* rather than being pressurized into doing so by someone else

 to follow my instructions in Part One *before* listening to the accompanying CD.

During the course of reading this book you will discover that I refer to cigarette smokers, when in fact you may be a pipe smoker or a cigar smoker. Naturally this treatment relates to every tobacco smoker. How you smoke the tobacco and the quantity you smoke make no difference to the outcome. You can become a non-smoker if you follow the instructions.

Also it may be necessary on certain occasions for me to repeat myself within this book; this not only helps to reinforce the messages but will ensure that anyone who is being selective and not reading the whole book before listening to the CD will receive the crucial messages.

I believe that we all have the right and freedom to choose whether to smoke or not. This book and CD are meant to help anyone who has decided that they would like to become a non-smoker.

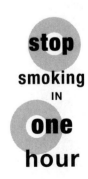

stop smoking IN one hour

I have been treating this problem for over 14 years and helping smokers to become non-smokers, working with both individuals and corporate clients. Through my research and experience with many thousands of delighted individuals, I have been able to put together this easy-to-follow book and CD package and explain to you exactly how you can become a non-smoker.

Part One will provide clear instructions to enable you to become a non-smoker. I will also endeavour to dispel any myths and fears that you may have regarding hypnosis, as there certainly is no need to feel anxious. I would like you to enter into this with a relaxed mind and without any traces of anxiety whatsoever regarding the method.

Part Two contains many useful and interesting facts, figures and government statistics – helpful if you feel the necessity to remind yourself why you have decided to become a non-smoker. It also contains many interesting comments from some of the delighted clients I have helped to become non-smokers during the last 14 years.

Part Two of this book can be read either before listening to the CD or afterwards. Although Part Two contains a tremendous amount of information, it is not critical to helping you to become a non-smoker, whereas Part One certainly is. In your eagerness to become a non-smoker, if you choose to read Part One only, before listening to the CD, please ensure that you read Part Two within a matter of days, as you will find it helpful in maintaining your resolve. In Part One you will read about the benefits of becoming a non-smoker, however you will not find any mention throughout my book of the benefits of being a smoker. There are NONE.

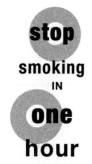

With this treatment it is important to understand that you are not 'giving something up' – so you won't feel deprived, or as though you

Cancer
and heart disease
are the two most common
fatal diseases.

Smoking is a major
cause of both.

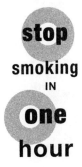

stop
smoking
IN
one
hour

Smoking Kills

It Is Not Selective

Smoking Can Kill Anyone

Smoking Can Kill You

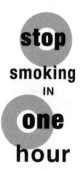

stop smoking IN **one** hour

are missing out on something, therefore you do not need a substitute. Instead, you will feel very proud of yourself because you are achieving something, achieving being a non-smoker, self-achievement. Enjoy that tremendous sense of pride and satisfaction. Just close your eyes when you are ready and take a few moments to allow that wonderful thought to float around inside your mind ... Think of someone offering you a cigarette and imagine yourself saying, 'No thank you, I don't smoke.'

When you 'give something up' (as with willpower alone and some other stop-smoking methods), you often feel deprived. If you experience a stressful day, you may think to yourself, 'Why have I given up smoking when I enjoy it?' (At stressful moments you will most probably have pleasurable memories of your smoking habit flooding back into your subconscious mind.)

We all have our own breaking point, and while there may be many days when you *almost* give in, you will decide to persevere after convincing yourself that you *can* do it this time.

If you do, however, decide to have a cigarette ... that first long, hard puff is heaven and you feel better, albeit for a short period...

BUT ... it is a myth to think that a cigarette will calm you.

The buzz that you experience with that first puff is short lived – around 7 seconds, to be precise – because as the reported 600 chemicals in tobacco smoke (which are irritants) enter the body, they act almost instantaneously as they come into contact with your brain, bronchial tubes, lungs and bloodstream. You feel irritable, more stressed, disappointed and at a loss to see how you can become a non-smoker. Also, whatever caused you to think you needed a cigarette in the first

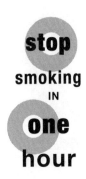

place (for example, stress or some problem) is still there and you still have to deal with it.

It may surprise you to know that it is the deep breath that you take in as you start a cigarette that causes the buzz and ensures instant gratification, *not* the cigarette. I will teach you breathing exercises during this treatment, which you will practise for three days following listening to the CD.

Let us not overlook the fact that if you do have that dreaded 'first cigarette' again (you will most probably have had many 'first cigarettes' in your smoking 'career'), as the realization that you have 'failed' hits you, you may experience thoughts of disbelief, self-disgust and disappointment – and so you start the cycle again of wanting to become a non-smoker.

I don't know about you, but that seems like purgatory to me. I would be thinking 'there must be an easier way.'

There *is* an easier way, which fortunately has been available for many years and therefore is well tried and tested.

This treatment is not a 'quick temporary fix'. It is permanent, can be very easy and allows you to remain calm and in control. Neither is it a hit-and-miss success; for every person who wishes to be a non-smoker for themselves they will achieve this, the easy way, using the 'Susan Hepburn formula'. Nor does it matter how many years you've been smoking, nor how many cigarettes (or how much tobacco in any form) you consume per day.

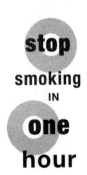

stop
smoking
IN
one
hour

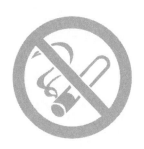

before

you

listen

to the

cd

you
can become
A non-smoker

When Is the Best Time to Become a Non-smoker?

The best time is when it feels right for you. There are many reasons why people smoke. Besides as a means to combat stress (though, as you will see, it is woefully inadequate for this), social and pleasurable times such as relaxing with your friends or family or having a drink often trigger smoking. Somehow the drink and cigarette go hand in hand, it seems you cannot have one without the other. This is purely a question of habit. In fact it is the relaxation and socializing that give you the enjoyment and buzz – certainly not the cigarettes. You only *think* it is the cigarettes.

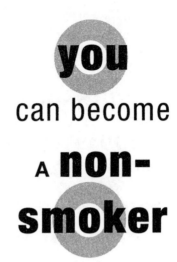

You can do whatever you **want** to do in life, providing it is **realistic**, if you think you can. It is mind over matter. **Believe** in yourself.

stop smoking IN **one** hour

With **your decision** to purchase this book and CD you have made a **huge** commitment to yourself and decided that the time is **right**, the **habit** must go.

You are one step closer to becoming a **non-smoker**.

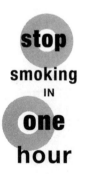

If you consider for a moment about yourself and your smoking habit ... when you light up a cigarette the first puff is a long, deep and slow draw, almost as if your life depended upon it or you cannot get enough of it. Subsequent puffs are shallow. The first puff gives you that tremendous surge of instant gratification as you take in a deep breath, then within seconds you continue smoking without a thought of what you are doing.

You most probably have asked yourself on many occasions when you are halfway through a cigarette, 'Why am I bothering to finish this?' Yet you invariably do, as a matter of habit.

You can become a non-smoker and you will become a non-smoker. This affirmation is not debatable but a fact, because *you* want to be a non-smoker.

There are no gimmicks to my treatment, just the simple fact that **you** wish to be a non-smoker. I repeat that I cannot do it for you. We are working together as a partnership. I am doing 80 per cent of the work and you are doing 20 per cent.

Without your contribution the treatment would not work. My contribution is that of a catalyst, putting the agreed suggestions (about your wish to become a non-smoker) into your subconscious mind so that you can act upon them. You have already contributed by committing yourself to becoming a non-smoker and purchasing this book and CD. The remainder of your contribution to this partnership consists of two further, easy commitments from you:

1. The desire to be a non-smoker for **yourself** first and foremost. There are always other reasons for wanting to become a non-smoker – financial considerations, health, a new baby in the family, a new partner who vehemently

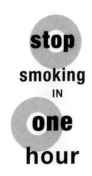

stop
smoking
IN
one
hour

opposes your smoking habit – but the most important factor has to be that **you** want to be a non-smoker for yourself. It is a most precious gift to yourself, from yourself: the gift of a proud, healthier and extended life.

 The commitment to engage in breathing exercises for three days following listening to the CD. The reasons for doing these exercises will become apparent later in this section. The breathing exercises are demonstrated clearly when you listen to the CD, however I would like you to give these exercises a try now.

👉 Breathing Exercises

Make sure that you are sitting comfortably. When you are ready, close your eyes and take a deep breath from your diaphragm. Hold that breath for a moment and then gradually let it out. Make this a movement that is easy for you to control. Carry on breathing deeply in and out, in and out.

Relax, but still let your mind and attention be concentrated on breathing. As you do so, realize that you are drawing in new life-force, new energy, for breath is life. Let this become an essence in your mind, wherever you are and whatever you are doing, realize that breath is life. Now continue with the breathing, gently in and out, approximately 12 times, in and out.

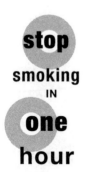

stop
smoking
IN
one
hour

I would like you to do the breathing exercises for three days following listening to the CD. Do them in the morning when you wake, then on the hour throughout the day and evening, and finally once more before you go to sleep. On each occasion breathe in and out approximately 12 times.

NOTE

If at any time during the three-day period you suddenly realize that you have forgotten to do the breathing exercises, for example for the past two or three hours, don't panic. This simply means that you did not feel the need to do them during that period. Do them as soon as you think of them again.

The benefits of the breathing exercises are twofold:

(1) When you take in a deep breath, you are taking oxygen into your lungs and into your bloodstream, thereby increasing the oxygen level. From the moment you smoke your last cigarette your body automatically begins to repair the damage they have done to you; the breathing exercises speed up this process. Also, if you think about it for a moment, when you take in a deep breath it is the same action as drawing on a cigarette/pipe/cigar, but this time you are taking in clean fresh oxygen instead of harmful chemicals and substances. When doing the breathing exercises you are imitating the action of smoking.

(2) The breathing exercises act like a trigger and a reminder of all the suggestions placed into your subconscious mind via the CD. If you *think* you want a cigarette – you do not want a cigarette, as you are a non-smoker – you are merely experiencing 'association'. A subconscious trigger will ensure that you instantly do your breathing exercises. The feeling of

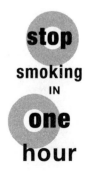

stop
smoking
IN
one
hour

need for a cigarette will go away in a matter of seconds. The chances of having to call upon these breathing exercises for this purpose are minimal, but you are now fully prepared and can use them if you need to.

The Importance of Practising the Breathing Exercises

I would like to explain to you how important the breathing exercises are, by using an analogy.

Let us assume that you decide to go to the gym, but as you have not been for some time you decide to invest in a personal fitness trainer to ensure that you know exactly what exercises to do, in order to obtain the maximum benefit. On completion of the training course you then go off to the gym on your own.

However, you decide after a few days that this seems too much like hard work and stop going to the gym. You would not expect your body to be toned, because you have not made the investment and therefore cannot expect a return. Very straightforward. You understand it is your own decision and will not begin to complain about it.

There is absolutely no excuse for failing to become a non-smoker with this treatment. Providing that you want to become a non-smoker _for yourself_, it can be very easy.

stop
smoking
IN
one
hour

Now I would like you to apply the same analogy to this treatment. I am the personal trainer for your mind and I will instruct you in the breathing exercises and explain their importance. If you invest, you will get a return. Practise the breathing exercises for three days following treatment, use the breathing exercises if ever you feel the need to smoke, and exercise your right to become a non-smoker the easy way. You will then enjoy a fitter, healthier and longer life. You have invested in the breathing exercises; your return is that you are a non-smoker.

Being a 'smoker' is NOT a prerequisite to enjoying life.

If you do feel the need to do the breathing exercises because you *think* you want a cigarette during the first two days following listening to the CD, they will help you reinforce the message that you are a non-smoker. The feeling is certainly not a desire or a craving for a cigarette, but merely association. It is crucial for you to understand this.

When I mention 'association' I am referring to the following experiences. How many of these are familiar and apply to you?

 The telephone rings and you reach for a cigarette.

 You cannot concentrate and you reach for a cigarette.

 Someone irritates you and you reach for a cigarette.

 A crisis happens and you reach for a cigarette.

 You're having a relaxing drink and you reach for a cigarette.

 After a meal, you have a cigarette.

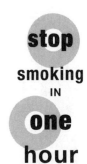

stop smoking IN one hour

Smoking **Kills**

It Is Not Selective

Smoking Can **Kill** Anyone

Smoking Can **Kill** You

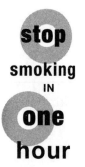

stop smoking IN one hour

You feel nervous before an interview/date/an important meeting, so you reach for a cigarette.

 The children have just gone to bed and you feel you deserve a reward, so you reach for a cigarette.

 You step out of an appointment with your dentist/doctor/lawyer and you reach for a cigarette.

 You step out of a 'non-smoking' environment such as the gym and you light a cigarette.

You do not need tobacco in order to be confident, cope with stress or enjoy life.

 At a party you accept every cigarette offered to you, have a sore throat the next morning and vow never to smoke again – until the next time!

Of course there are many more of these 'associations'. You could undoubtedly add to the list yourself. However, you have one main reason for becoming a non-smoker: *you* have decided to become a non-smoker and the time is right.

NOTE
When you have completed the treatment you are a non-smoker – but remember, you are a *new* non-smoker.

If you experience 'association' and possibly second thoughts as to why you are putting yourself through what you deem to be unnecessary

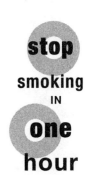

stop
smoking
IN
one
hour

suffering (in fact these thoughts are just an excuse to have a cigarette), then do the breathing exercises and remind yourself exactly why you decided to embark upon this treatment.

NOTE

If anyone is vulnerable it is usually during the first two days, so please remain aware. Also, if you do experience any difficulties, remember that these are not cravings but merely associations. They will not be as severe as 'withdrawal symptoms' (which you may have previously experienced). Persevere and remain positive and confident about your success. You can do it. This mental preparation and attitude are exactly what's required to ensure your success in becoming a non-smoker.

Do not leave your future in the hands of the tobacco companies. They need you. You do not need them.

If you're still worried about your chances of success, be reassured by the most common comments made to me over the years:

 'I cannot believe how easy it has been'.

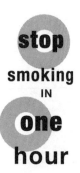

 'Is there a catch to this, because even though I have not had a cigarette, nor do I want a cigarette, when anyone offers me one I am saying that I don't smoke? It is strange but wonderful'.

'I never really believed that I would become a non-smoker, as I have been smoking for over 20 years and tried so many times before.'

'It was so easy to stop smoking. I became worried it would wear off. You took away the pain. I don't know how it works or why it works, it just does and I am very happy.'

'Even though I know you said that we would work together as a partnership, I really felt that I did no work at all, it was *so* easy.'

Many clients over the years comment that they cannot even remember what it felt like to smoke.

At this stage I would suggest you make a list of the reasons why you have decided to become a non-smoker; it can be handy to refer to during the first two days after you have listened to the CD, if you feel the need.

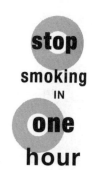

The reasons could include some or all of the following:

 Becoming a non-smoker reduces the risk of over 50 different illnesses and conditions.

 I will be healthier and live longer.

 The risk of a heart attack falls to the same as that of a non-smoker within 10–15 years.

 The risk of developing lung cancer is only slightly greater than that of a lifelong non-smoker within 10–15 years.[1]

 The cancer risk drops with every year of not smoking.

 I will be a role model for children, both my own and other people's.

 I will be able to climb stairs without getting out of breath.

 My fitness will be improved and I will be able to participate in more sporting activities.

 I will have a better chance of having a healthy baby.

 Food and drink will taste better as my taste buds will be cleaner.

 My skin will be clean and my complexion will be clearer.

 My breath, hair and clothes will be fresher, and there'll be no more cigarette smells around the house.

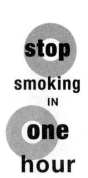
stop
smoking
IN
one
hour

I will no longer be the tool of the tobacco companies. **15**

 I will be making a contribution to the health of the environment.

 I will definitely enjoy having more money to spend.

Since your smoking 'career' began you have probably stopped and started again and again, always knowing in the back of your mind that when you had 'succeeded' it was really just a temporary interlude and that you would eventually return to smoking.

From the moment you finish listening to this CD you can become a non-smoker. Thousands of satisfied non-smokers know it works.

Since you had your first cigarette you have not experienced life without cigarettes; such a life has become unknown territory.

There have been very few smokers in my experience who have never attempted to become non-smokers. Indeed, you may be one of the many smokers who are so pleased with yourself for 'stopping smoking' for several weeks or even months, so delighted because you have saved lots of money and given your lungs a rest, that you decide to reward yourself ... with a cigarette! After all, it was so easy quitting, you could always do it again, right?

This time is different. You somehow know that it is different, you know that 'this is it,' no more smoking. How does that make you feel?

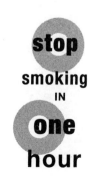

stop smoking IN one hour

To some people this comes as a huge relief, but to others it seems like a tremendous responsibility and they think, 'How will I cope?'

You can do
whatever you want
to do in life if you think
you can. Self-achievement
is mind over matter.

Believe in yourself.

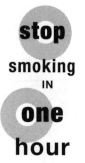

stop
smoking
IN
one
hour

You will cope, absolutely. It is as easy as you make it. Demonstrate your commitment using this method and you will succeed and feel very proud of yourself.

Remember it was not curiosity that prompted you to purchase this book and CD, but your commitment and determination. When you have got this far, the next and final step is easy.

Another reminder for those of you who feel you need cigarettes in order to have fun or relax: It is the social aspect that is enjoyable, *not* the cigarettes. With every smoker there will usually be a memory of times when you have felt desperate for a cigarette, before an interview perhaps. You have little time to spare for that cigarette but you think you desperately need one and, panicking now, this thought crosses your mind: 'What if the interview goes on longer than expected and I need a cigarette?' A few quick puffs are required, and you stand there drawing frantically on the cigarette, but do you enjoy it? ... I doubt it.

You can now put all of these embarrassing and desperate incidents behind you.

You were born with self-confidence, self-assuredness and self-assertiveness. This wonderful package of positive emotions is part of you, yet as you grow through childhood, your early teens, right through to now, any one of these positive emotions can be attacked and eroded away, a little at a time.

Each time that you experience trauma, whether it be minor or major, these positive emotions are attacked and eroded away. Nevertheless, they remain part of you, lying dormant within you.

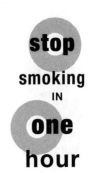

stop
smoking
IN
one
hour

18

When listening to the CD I will make you aware of and help you to rediscover these emotions, to reclaim your own natural inner strength and inner resources, the tools of life which enable you to deal with life's problems in a most efficient and effective manner. And one of these problems is that you are a smoker and wish to become a non-smoker. **You can and you will**, from the moment that you finish listening to the CD.

Finally, and most important of all, you must want to achieve this ideal of becoming a non-smoker, you must want it *for yourself*, you must want it very badly.

By becoming a non-smoker:

 You have embarked upon a self-improvement programme and taken the first and most major step towards a healthier, better and longer life.

 You will become more confident and feel better about yourself.

 Your energy levels will increase enormously and you will perform better at physical activities.

 You will be fitter and therefore enjoy life more.

 Your increased confidence will enable you to deal with stress more effectively and efficiently.

 You will feel very proud of yourself and have a tremendous sense of well-being.

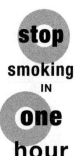 You will enjoy a healthier looking complexion, healthier hair, and clothes that smell fresh.

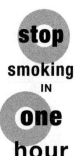

Final Preparations for Becoming a Non-smoker

Each smoker who has made the commitment to become a non-smoker by listening to the CD that comes with this book prepares in a different way.

This treatment is not a quick temporary fix – it is permanent.

Some feel that they need a final cigarette as a way of saying goodbye to an old pal, a faithful 'friend' (although it is certainly a false one, one you are much better off without), just before listening to the CD.

Others surprise themselves by discovering that they are already keen to become non-smokers from the moment they start reading this book. Although they may have intended to have a final cigarette, they choose not to.

There are also those who will have chosen a particular date on which to become a non-smoker, even if they have bought the book and CD days before. They smoke their last cigarette the night before and listen to the CD first thing next morning. However, they will not entertain the idea of a cigarette that day if circumstances dictate that they have to listen to the CD later in the day. The date has been set in their minds, and for them has to be a 'smoke-free' day and the first of a lifetime of 'smoke-free' days.

There are still others, albeit very few, who want to smoke as many cigarettes as possible before they embark on the final part of this treatment (listening to the CD). I recall one gentleman at my clinic

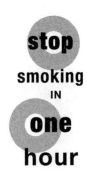
stop smoking IN **one hour**

**You can beat
the smoking habit here and
now after listening to the CD.**

Enjoy being a non-smoker.

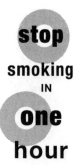

stop
smoking
IN
one
hour

several years ago, who smoked *40* cigarettes *before* our 10 a.m. appointment. But he really was an exception. I wondered what time he must have got up that morning in order to smoke such a vast amount! I told him that he might have to work harder with his breathing exercises, but was highly delighted to discover that he had joined the happy band of non-smokers. Incidentally, he returned several months later to master his fear of flying.

I would like to reassure you that of the aforementioned methods of preparation there is not one that is better than the others or indeed the 'right' way. The method that suits you is always the best one, the right one for you.

Think Positive – Remain Committed to Becoming a Non-smoker

If this is not the first time you have tried to achieve the wonderful, healthy state of being a non-smoker, then you will know that, on your own, it can be difficult and is inevitably short-lived. With this treatment it can be easy.

The permanence is due partly to the fact that with this treatment you are not giving something up, so you do not feel deprived, you do not feel that you are missing out on anything. You feel proud, you feel very proud of yourself because you are achieving something, you are achieving being a non-smoker. You think of yourself as a non-smoker because that is exactly what you are, so why would you ever think of having a cigarette? You won't. Smoking is no longer worthy of the energy of your thought process.

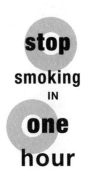

stop
smoking
IN
one
hour

listening
to the
cd

To gain maximum benefit from the CD you must find the right time for you, 30 minutes when you can relax totally. Select a time and place where you know that you can remain at peace and not be disturbed for the duration of this 30-minute CD. As a smoker you will understand that these 30 minutes will prove vital for a healthier, longer life and freedom, so be prepared to wait until you can give the best 30 minutes of your attention. You will instinctively know when the time is right.

When you have chosen your 'quality 30 minutes' and have therefore decided that you are ready to become a non-smoker, close the curtains, dim the lights and silence the telephone. Relax and enjoy.

NOTE
If you have children, ensure that they are either in bed, at school or being taken care of by someone, to avoid any possible distractions.

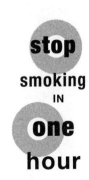

stop
smoking
IN
one
hour

Make yourself comfortable and warm (it is easier to relax in a warm room). I would advise you to lie down on or in your bed or on a comfy sofa (cover yourself with a warm throw). Spend some time making sure that the volume on the CD is perfect for you (fairly low but pleasantly audible – too low and you are straining to hear, too high and it can appear intrusive).

While listening to my voice you will enjoy a pleasurable experience as you are able to release all the tensions from your body and drift into a most beautiful state of total, complete and utter relaxation.

When you begin listening to the CD, make sure that you are comfortable and have taken the necessary precautions as outlined previously to ensure that you are not going to be disturbed. Throughout the recording listen very carefully, giving it your full attention. It is a pleasure to be enjoyed and to look forward to.

I will guide you into the hypnotic state, which is a state of total relaxation within the body and a state of increased and heightened awareness within the mind so you hear everything I say to you.

The hypnotic state is similar to when you are drifting off to sleep at night, when you are neither fully awake nor asleep and are aware of familiar noises in the background. Anything unfamiliar causes you to become immediately alert and ready to deal with the situation.

stop
smoking
IN
one
hour

Therefore if you are listening to the CD and the doorbell rings or something else demands your immediate attention, you will be able to open your eyes and deal with the situation without any ill-effects whatsoever. If this should happen or if you are distracted for any other reason, when you are ready to listen to the CD again please start from the beginning, in order to allow yourself to relax totally and to ensure optimum benefit.

During the state of hypnosis, thoughts and ideas may enter your mind. For example, you may experience thoughts that are completely unconnected to smoking. This is perfectly natural; please do not let it concern you. When you enter the hypnotic state the mind is in a state of heightened awareness, so is more open to outside stimuli and distractions.

The breathing exercises demonstrated at the beginning of the CD will help you to clear your mind of any irrelevancies of the day, to relieve your body of all tension and to help you concentrate your mind on entering the hypnotic state and becoming a non-smoker.

Tips for Becoming a Non-smoker

S tart with a firm plan and set a date to become a non-smoker, then look forward to that date.

T hink about why you have decided to become a non-smoker and make a list of your reasons. Then if you ever feel tempted to have a cigarette, remind yourself why you became a non-smoker and read your list.

O nly become a non-smoker if you are convinced it is something that you want to do for yourself, rather than being pressurized into doing so from someone else and ensure the time is right for you.

P leasure – think of the pleasure when you are offered a cigarette and you are able to say, 'no thank you I don't smoke.'

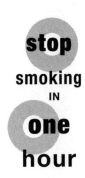

stop
smoking
IN
one
hour

the
benefits
of becoming a
non-smoker

Smoking kills more than 120,000 people every year in Britain, and 480,000 people in the US.[2]

Smoking is the leading preventable cause of death, yet so many thousands every year start smoking. Why do they do it? The same reasons you did.

We owe it to our ourselves and to future generations to become non-smokers, to understand that we can cope perfectly well without tobacco and enjoy life more without it. The dependency that you have experienced has been psychological rather than physical. It may have seemed difficult in the past to become a non-smoker, but with this method you will not only enjoy the treatment but will also be pleasantly surprised at how easily you can become a non-smoker.

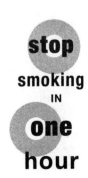

stop
smoking
IN
one
hour

Tobacco is a uniquely dangerous product.

If introduced today, it would not stand the remotest chance of being legalized.

But smoking is not against the law.

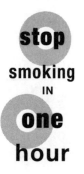

stop
smoking
IN
one
hour

When smokers are confronted with the harsh reality of the problems – both health-related and social – that their smoking habit brings for themselves and others, the majority admit that they have always intended to become non-smokers, but that there has always been an excuse to put it off to a 'better' time.

All smokers' energy levels are depleted because of lack of oxygen in the bloodstream. Oxygen levels decrease by about 15 per cent when smoking, to be replaced by carbon monoxide. When you become a non-smoker your energy levels will increase and your senses will be heightened, especially your sense of taste and sense of smell as your nasal passages clear.

To ensure success it is crucial to have a positive attitude, to mentally prepare and convince yourself that you will succeed.

I have always believed that the transition from being a smoker to a non-smoker should be as smooth and uneventful as possible. Why remind yourself each day that you used to smoke, or feel the need to congratulate yourself for getting through another day without tobacco? Far better just to forget you ever were a smoker. And with this method, you will eventually forget you were a smoker.

No more embarrassment when you have told all your friends and family that you are a non-smoker, only to announce later that you are smoking again, resulting in yet another blow to your self-esteem.

You can become a non-smoker if you are given the right tools to do so.

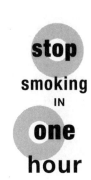

stop smoking IN **one hour**

Every day over 1,000 adults in the UK become non-smokers, which equates to over 350,000 every year. A similar percentage of US smokers (some 3 per cent) kick the habit every year.

 With a positive attitude and the right mental preparation, you will be one of them.

When you become a non-smoker, both men and women experience significant and immediate health benefits. The body systems begin to return to normal and the body immediately begins to repair the damage.

Time Since Quitting	Effects[3]
20 minutes	Blood pressure and pulse rate return to normal. Circulation improves, making you look healthier as well as feel healthier.
8 hours	Nicotine and carbon monoxide levels in the blood are greatly reduced; oxygen levels in the blood return to normal. The chances of a heart attack start to fall.
24 hours	Carbon monoxide is eliminated from the body. Lungs start to clear out mucus and other smoking debris.
48 hours	Nicotine has been eliminated from the body. Your senses of taste and smell are greatly enhanced.
72 hours	Bronchial tubes begin to relax; energy levels increase. Breathing becomes easier.

stop
smoking
IN
one
hour

2 – 12 weeks	Circulation improves throughout the body.
3 – 9 months	Lung function is increased by up to 10 per cent, therefore coughing, wheezing and breathing problems improve.
5 years	Risk of heart attack falls to approximately half that of a smoker.
10 years	Risk of lung cancer falls to half that of a smoker. Risk of heart attack falls to the same as for someone who has never smoked.

You do not need a cigarette (pipe, cigar, etc.) to relax or to enjoy life. Smoking only *appears* to reduce the tension created by the habit. BUT ... the reported 600 chemicals in tobacco smoke are irritants, therefore they cannot relax you. It is the act of taking in a deep breath when drawing on a cigarette that is the relaxant. This is, however, only short-lived (lasting about 7 seconds). Very quickly the relaxed state is followed by the chemicals entering the brain, lungs, bronchial tubes, bloodstream, etc. and causing irritation.

I would like you to forget you were a smoker, and you can.

To relax we all need to inhale pure, life-giving air, hold it in for a few moments, and then exhale. Breath is life; pure breath is healthier, longer life.

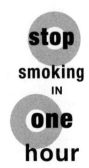

stop smoking IN one hour

No cigarette ...

deep rhythmic breathing ...

perfect relaxation.

Every time.

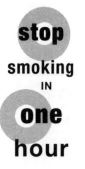

stop
smoking
IN
one
hour

As a smoker you will undoubtedly have experienced inner conflicts regarding whether you wish to become a non-smoker or not. Have you experienced a severe cold, influenza or chest infection and seriously thought about becoming a non-smoker, but have always found an excuse not to do so? There will most probably have been days when you have thought of little else other than, 'I really must stop smoking.'

Conversely, you will probably be familiar with the following argument: 'I enjoy smoking, so why should I give it up?' These inner conflicts exist within most smokers, the battle between knowing that you want to, must or ought to become a non-smoker and the fact that you enjoy *certain* cigarettes. (In my experience I have never treated anyone who admits to enjoying *every* cigarette.) Occasionally I have treated someone who has said 'I would give everything I have to become a non-smoker,' and some who have said, 'I really hate smoking,' but they have also been exceptions to the rule.

Very occasionally when smokers first arrive in my consulting room they are feeling anxious at becoming non-smokers, and utter reservations that not only do they enjoy some of their cigarettes but also that they are afraid of being without cigarettes. These clients have usually made previous attempts to become non-smokers, with dreadful withdrawal symptoms.

One of my priorities with all my clients is to explain fully how the method works and to allay any of their fears. I shall do that with you also before you listen to the CD.

Through hypnosis we are able to locate and bring back to the forefront of the mind those time-worn positive emotions that have been suppressed. When we attempt a task and fail, our negative emotions

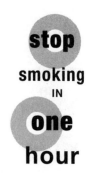

You will eventually forget you were a smoker.

Why would you wish to remember?

Why should becoming a non-smoker be difficult?

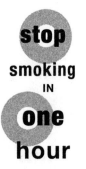

stop
smoking
IN
one
hour

suppress our self-confidence, self-esteem and self-assurance. So if we fail the first time we are more likely to fail the second time and the third time and so on ...

With the help of hypnotherapy we are able to return to the first time, to complete the task and succeed, for example by taking control of your smoking habit and becoming a non-smoker.

Words to the Wise

You might want to take note of these useful reminders:

 One of the fundamental requirements for my treatment to be effective is your desire to be a non-smoker. We work together as a partnership. I am the catalyst, putting the agreed suggestions into your subconscious mind. You act upon them. You have to play your part in this treatment; I cannot do it for you.

 The major hurdles associated with becoming a non-smoker – the misconception that you will eat more and the notion that you will suffer terrible 'withdrawal symptoms' – are dealt with in my treatment and will therefore not be an issue.

 On completion of the treatment, when you become a non-smoker, enjoy – but be aware. If anyone is ever vulnerable it is usually during the first two days, so if you feel irritated for whatever reason and think you want a cigarette, remember that you are irritated with life's problems and frustrations.

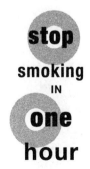

You have not changed, life is always going to throw up problems and frustrations, whether you smoke or not. Do your breathing exercises and the urge for a cigarette will go away almost instantly (in a matter of seconds rather than minutes).

 Beware of smokers who will offer you a cigarette, saying 'Just the one won't hurt.' Well, one *will* hurt and will completely undo what you have finally achieved.

 The success of hypnosis is not hit-and-miss. It works for every person who wants to be a non-smoker. It doesn't matter how many years you've smoked nor how many cigarettes (or how much tobacco) you smoke per day.

 The treatment is not a quick temporary fix. It is permanent.

 A crucial key to success with any hypnotherapy treatment lies in the client and hypnotherapist working together as a partnership.

 You have an expectation and belief that you are going to succeed in becoming a non-smoker. This can only happen if you understand and undertake your role in the treatment. There is inevitably someone now and again who believes that they can hand over full responsibility to the hypnotherapist. This is a misconception. I would like to do it for you, as I am sure most hypnotherapists would, but it cannot be done. I am dealing with your mind and could not make you do anything that you don't want to. You have to want to be a non-smoker for the treatment to succeed, and you have to want this for yourself.

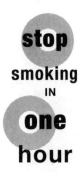

stop
smoking
IN
one
hour

When in the hypnotic state you hear everything that is said and do not relinquish control to the hypnotherapist at any time.

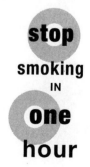

hypnosis:
frequently
asked
questions

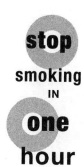

What is Hypnosis?

Hypnosis is a natural state of total relaxation within the body and a state of increased awareness within the mind. As you enter the hypnotic state you will become less aware of your surroundings and more aware of your inner feelings. You will automatically focus your attention on the suggestions that are being put to you, in order to master a particular problem. The suggestions are always agreed beforehand and are suggestions that you want to be made.

During hypnosis you are in an altered state of consciousness where changes can easily be made to induce healing, increase self-awareness and access many more positive assertions.

**stop
smoking
IN
one
hour**

During hypnosis you
are neither asleep
nor fully awake and you
do not relinquish control
at any time.

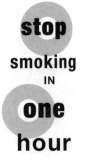

stop
smoking
IN
one
hour

In this relaxed state the subconscious part of the mind is more receptive and therefore able to respond to outside stimuli and suggestions. The suggestions concern areas that you would like to change about yourself.

What Is Hypnotherapy?

Hypnotherapy uses hypnosis to facilitate change. Agreed positive suggestions are placed into the subconscious level of your mind while you are in the relaxed state of hypnosis. The suggestions are your conscious desires, for example that you have no cravings or desire to smoke. During hypnosis you will never act upon any suggestions that you do not agree with.

What If I Cannot Be Hypnotized?

Anyone can be hypnotized providing that they *want* to be. The exceptions are, for example, those who are influenced by alcohol or illegal drugs, in which case the therapist would not even attempt to hypnotize them.

The fact that you have purchased this book and CD demonstrates that you are willing to be hypnotized. Please be aware that you will not feel as you expect to feel during the hypnotic state. The expectation is usually that you will be asleep and not aware of anything going on around you, but the opposite is true. You are fully aware throughout and could easily stop the session at any time.

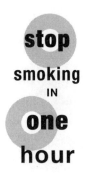

stop
smoking
IN
one
hour

Will I Remember What Has Been Said to Me?

The majority of clients remember everything that is said to them during hypnosis, as they are in a state of increased awareness. The hypnotic state is very similar to the way you feel just before falling asleep, when you're totally relaxed but fully aware of everything around you. You are neither asleep nor fully awake. If there were familiar noises you would happily continue going to sleep, however if there were unfamiliar noises you would open your eyes and deal with the situation – the hypnotic state is very similar, as you hear everything around you.

How Will I Feel During Hypnosis?

You will feel pleasantly relaxed, as though you are in a trance-like, dreamy state. Feelings of euphoria are common, but you are unlikely to feel 'hypnotized'. Most people have expressed a sense of 'waiting for it to happen' and usually think that they will be asleep during the hypnotic state, but, as I have said, the opposite is true. During hypnosis you are in a state of increased awareness.

Prepare yourself mentally ... remember that you are not alone. The majority of smokers would like to quit, and about 3 million attempt each year in the UK.

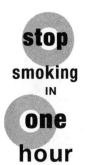

stop
smoking
IN
one
hour

You may experience bodily changes as you enter the hypnotic state. Your body may feel unusually light or unusually heavy, and sometimes there can be a strange sense as though you cannot feel your body at all. You could even experience a combination of two of these sensations or of all three, or a warm tingling in the hands or feet. This is due to the transition from the conscious state to the subconscious state and the release of tensions from your body. Whatever you experience it is perfectly natural and always a most pleasant experience.

You may feel as though you do not want to move even though you know you can, because you have a sense of coming out of the pleasant relaxed state that you are in and do not wish to do so. Time will appear to pass very quickly.

You will experience Rapid Eye Movement (REM) as you enter the hypnotic state, and therefore may have a sensation of the eyelids flickering, although most people are not aware of this sensation.

How Does Hypnosis Work?

Agreed suggestions are placed into your subconscious mind to help you to overcome problems. In this instance, suggestions will be placed into your subconscious mind that you have no cravings for tobacco, no desire to eat more, no bad temper or irritability and no concern that you are missing out on anything, so will not feel deprived or in need of a substitute. The hypnotic suggestions are only effective if you allow them to be.

Can Anyone Be Hypnotized?

Yes, providing that the circumstances are right, as explained earlier (so long as the person is not under the influence of alcohol or drugs), and providing you want to be hypnotized. If you are undergoing hypnosis because someone else has pressurized you into trying it, then it will not work.

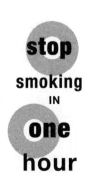

stop smoking IN **one hour**

Are There Any Adverse Side-effects to Hypnosis?

No. Hypnosis is used to facilitate positive change. You are in complete control throughout the hypnotic state. The benefits of hypnosis can be felt immediately.

You cannot be made to do anything that you do not want to do and will not accept any suggestions which would not be acceptable to your conscious mind.

Will You Make Me Do Silly Things?

No, you would never do or say anything while in the hypnotic state which you would not normally do and in particular which goes against your moral code. It is only the stage hypnotist who will encourage people to do silly things, but this is for entertainment value only. Usually the participants have an idea of the tasks that they will be asked to perform before going on stage, and are therefore prepared to do silly things. In this instance you are listening to the CD for therapeutic reasons; there is no need to have you behave in any way that is silly or 'entertaining'.

Will I Lose Control During the Session?

stop smoking IN one hour

No, you do not relinquish control whatsoever. You are in complete control throughout and can stop the session at any time. You will be fully aware and hear everything that is said to you, as you are in a state of increased awareness. A hypnotherapist can never gain control over your mind but will assist you, through suggestions, to take control of your life and the habits that you wish to change.

You will. You can open your eyes at any time during the session, ending the hypnotic state immediately. You can do this at any time you wish to, as you are in complete control throughout. I will guide you into the hypnotic state and continue guiding you throughout the treatment, but whether you choose to follow is entirely up to you.

When you are listening to the CD you can return to full consciousness immediately if you need to (if the doorbell rings, for instance), without any ill effects whatsoever. If you listen to the CD as you go to bed you will most probably drift into a natural sleep (after you have finished listening to the CD) and awaken the next morning feeling refreshed, having recharged your batteries.

How Will I Feel After the Hypnosis?

Most people feel very relaxed and quite sleepy following hypnosis, and have been known to fall asleep more easily than usual that night. Others feel exceptionally happy. All feel energetic the following day – this is due in part to increased oxygen levels in the bloodstream.

Becoming a Non-smoker

Most find that becoming a non-smoker with this treatment is incredibly easy, however for the few who do experience difficulties it can seem like a long struggle. As a 'struggler' you may feel restless and frustrated, but persevere because you will experience these emotions for only two or three days. Then you will quickly begin to feel the benefits of becoming a non-smoker and rejoice in your sheer determination to succeed.

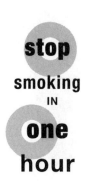

Consider for a moment what you could do with the money that you spend on cigarettes ... main brand cigarettes currently cost over £4 a pack in the UK, and nearly $4 in the US. The table below shows how much smoking costs at current prices in the UK and US.

Cigarettes per day	Over 1 year (UK/US)	5 years	10 years	20 years	50 years
10	£730/$640	£3,650/$3,200	£7,300/$6,400	£14,600/$12,800	£36,500/$32,000
20	£1,460/$1,280	£7,300/$6,400	£14,600/$12,800	£29,200/$25,600	£73,000/$64,000
40	£2,920/$2,560	£14,600/$12,800	£29,200/$25,600	£58,400/$51,200	£146,000/$128,000

Name the Day

Choose a date to become a non-smoker. Some would make it a New Year's resolution, many choose Monday mornings, while for others their birthday or 'National No Smoking Day' (an annual event in the UK, held the second Wednesday in March) or 'American Smoke-Out Day' (organized by the American Lung Association in March every year) is the day for them. Having a particular day to focus on will help with your mental preparation.

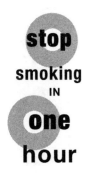

stop
smoking
IN
one
hour

Demonstrate commitment and determination ... it is important to be committed to becoming a non-smoker and to avoid the common error of not taking the matter seriously. Face the challenge with determination, you cannot afford to allow cigarettes to control you ever again.

Decide to become a non-smoker in one hit ... although in theory it may seem easier to reduce the number of cigarettes smoked each day, when the time comes to relinquish those last two or three cigarettes, you'll find you're not prepared to go this final step. This method is virtually impossible to sustain because, as you cut down each day, the likelihood is that you will smoke every cigarette more intensively and can begin to feel deprived. The best approach is to go for a complete break.

Now you are prepared mentally and emotionally to listen to the accompanying CD. Make space and time for yourself (as discussed on page 23), relax and feel secure in the knowledge that very soon you will be a non-smoker!

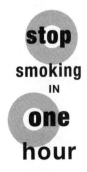

stop
smoking
IN
one
hour

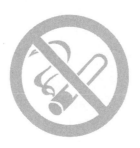

after the cd:

facts, figures and

case studies

to help

you stay

smoke-free

passive
smoking

Passive smoking (exposure to other people's tobacco smoke) consists of:

sidestream smoke – smoke from the burning end of the cigarette

mainstream smoke – smoke inhaled and exhaled by the smoker

environmental tobacco smoke (ETS) – a combination of sidestream and mainstream smoke and a major source of indoor pollution

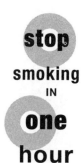

stop
smoking
IN
one
hour

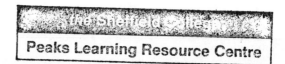

It is estimated that passive smoking causes several hundred cases of lung cancer and several thousand cases of heart disease in non-smokers in the UK every year.

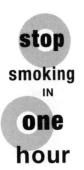

stop
smoking
IN
one
hour

The US Environmental Protection Agency has declared passive smoking or exposure to environmental tobacco smoke (ETS) to be a 'Class A Carcinogen', which means that it is capable of causing cancer in humans.[4]

This section may seem filled with doom and gloom, and I apologize in advance if I cause irritation and cries of, 'Well, they *would* say that, wouldn't they?' ('they' being non-smokers), but it is essential to make smokers aware of the reasons why a non-smoker may seem to over-react when anyone lights a cigarette within close proximity. It is also reasonable to inform non-smokers about all the dangers of passive smoking and, finally, to help you to become aware of the dangers of passive smoking because you are about to become a non-smoker.

Evidence of the health impact of passive smoking has been building up over the past two decades, including that found in reports from the UK Independent Scientific Committee on Smoking and Health, the US National Research Council and the National and Medical Research Council of Australia.[5]

Over the past two years, further major reviews on passive smoking have been published. These include studies by the UK Government-appointed Scientific Committee on Tobacco and Health,[6] a World Health Organization Consultation report on ETS and Child Health[7] and a report by the California Environmental Protection Agency (EPA)[8]. All the studies identified passive smoking as a risk factor for the following:

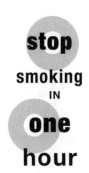

stop
smoking
IN
one
hour

Illnesses in Adults Caused by Passive Smoking

 lung cancer

 ischaemic heart disease

 reduced lung function in adults with no chronic chest problems

 increased sensitivity and reduced lung function in asthmatics

 irritation of the eyes, nose and throat

 aggravation of allergies

 increased risk of stroke

 nasal cancer

 cervical cancer

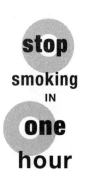

In the US, 3,000
Americans die every year
of lung cancer, while a further
134,000 die of heart disease
(this includes all heart disease
deaths – both those caused
by ETS and those caused
by smoking).[9]

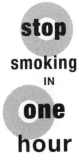

Illnesses in Babies and Young Children Caused by Passive Smoking

 increased risk of lower respiratory tract infection

 increased severity of asthma symptoms

 more frequent occurrence of chronic coughs, phlegm and wheezing

 low birthweight problems

 increased risk of cot death (SIDS)

 chronic middle ear infection

 bronchitis

 pneumonia

 cancers and leukaemia

 meningococcal infections

More than 17,000 children under the age of five are admitted to hospital every year in the UK because of the effects of passive smoking. Some 300,000 children in the US suffer from lower respiratory tract infections every year, again caused by passive smoking.[10]

And it's worth remembering that, unlike adults, young children do not have any choice regarding their exposure to passive smoking.

Research analysing 37 published epidemiological studies of the risk of lung cancer in non-smokers (4,626 cases in all) found that the risk of lung cancer in life-long non-smokers who lived with a smoker was 24 per cent.[11] Any adjustment for factors such as diet had little overall effect.

Tobacco-specific carcinogens in the blood of non-smokers provided clear evidence of the effect of passive smoking.

The authors concluded that 'non-smokers exposed to environmental tobacco smoke (ETS), provides compelling confirmation that breathing other people's tobacco smoke is a cause of lung cancer.'

A major European study of non-smokers exposed to ETS, who lived with smokers or worked in a smoky environment, were also found to have an increased risk of lung cancer, in the region of 20–30 per cent.[12]

This extensive study was conducted in 12 centres within 7 European countries using 650 patients with lung cancer and 1,542 subjects up to 74 years of age.

The subjects were asked about their exposure to ETS during childhood, adulthood, at home, in the workplace, in vehicles and in public places.

The study found that exposure during childhood was not associated with an increased risk of lung cancer.

Passive Smoking and Heart Disease

Studies in the early 1990s estimated that heart disease caused by passive smoking was the third leading preventable cause of death in the US, ranking behind active smoking and alcohol abuse.[13] The study also demonstrated that non-smokers living with smokers long term had about a 30 per cent increased risk of heart disease.

Since then, further studies have shown conclusively that exposure to ETS increases the risk of heart disease in non-smokers. It would appear that even a low-level exposure to tobacco smoke has a profound effect on heart disease, because exposure to ETS causes the blood to thicken – a phenomenon known as platelet aggregation.

The studies concluded that, unlike the risk for lung cancer which is roughly in proportion to smoke exposure, passive smokers' risk of heart disease may be as much as half that of someone smoking 20 cigarettes a day, even though they would only inhale about 1 per cent of the smoke.

A review of 19 published studies of 'the risk of heart disease and non-smokers' found that non-smokers have an overall 23 per cent increased risk of heart disease when living with a smoker.[14]

stop
smoking
IN
one
hour

Further studies revealed that while the risk of heart disease in non-smokers exposed to ETS is proportionally large, some of the early damage to arteries caused by passive smoking may be reversible in healthy adults if further tobacco smoke is avoided for at least a year.[15] The studies also found that an even greater improvement in former passive smokers was evident after two years of cessation of passive smoking.

Research in New Zealand revealed that exposure to passive smoking increased the risk of strokes in non-smokers by 82 per cent.[16] By comparison, active smokers had a fourfold risk of stroke compared with people who had never smoked or had stopped smoking more than 10 years earlier and who were not exposed to ETS. Given that a stroke is a common condition, this indicates quite clearly that passive smoking is having a serious health impact on non-smokers.

Passive Smoking and Respiratory Disease

Passive smoking has subtle but significant effects on the respiratory health of non-smoking adults, including increased coughing, phlegm production, chest discomfort and reduced lung function.

There are 3.5 million asthma sufferers in the UK, and ETS causes difficulties for 80 per cent of them.[17]

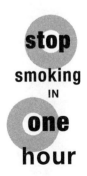

vital statistics:

THE STARK

realities of smoking

We cannot afford to underestimate the dangers of smoking and it is with this in mind that I sought the permission of ASH (Action on Smoking and Health) and the UK Government Health Education Authority to include the following statistics in this book. I also appreciate the opportunity to assist these organizations in creating an awareness of the effects of smoking.

The statistics make alarming reading but we cannot and must not ignore them. As you will discover throughout this book, passive smoking carries dangers; we can only thank ASH and the government for their interminable quest to ensure teenagers are made aware of the grave dangers of smoking, to ensure many public places become smoke free zones and to be instrumental in banning tobacco advertising, to name but a few of their aims.

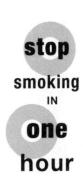

stop
smoking
IN
one
hour

Approximately
half of all regular
cigarette smokers
will eventually be killed
by their habit.[18]

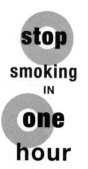

stop
smoking
IN
one
hour

There are over 12 million smokers in the UK, over one-quarter of the adult population – 29 per cent of men and 28 per cent of women. In the US this figure stands at 48.5 million (26.5 million men and 22 million women above 18 years of age, which includes 1.5 million female adolescents).

30 per cent of all cancer deaths can be attributed to smoking. Cancers other than lung cancer which are linked to smoking include:

 cancers of the mouth and lip

 cervical cancer

 liver cancer

 cancer of the pancreas

 cancer of the kidney

 bladder cancer

 stomach cancer

 cancer of the oesophagus

 nose and throat cancer

 cancer of the larynx

 leukaemia

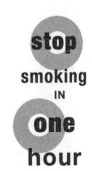

Smoking and Lung Cancer

Intensive epidemiological studies in the UK and US have proved beyond any shadow of doubt that cigarette smoking markedly increases the chances of developing lung cancer.[19]

Smoking causes around 82 per cent of all deaths from lung cancer.

Smokers who smoke between 1 and 14 cigarettes a day have 8 times the risk of dying from lung cancer compared to non-smokers.

Smokers who smoke more than 25 cigarettes a day have 25 times the risk of dying from lung cancer compared to non-smokers.

Smoking and Heart Disease

Smoking causes around 25 per cent of all deaths in the UK from heart disease. In the US this figure rises to 50 per cent, taking in all cases of hypertension (high blood pressure) and strokes.

Cigarette smoking increases the risk of having a heart attack by two to three times, compared with the risk to non-smokers.

About 90 per cent of cases of peripheral vascular disease, which leads to amputation of one or both legs, are caused by smoking – about 2,000 amputations a year.

Smoking and Respiratory Diseases

It is reported that 83 per cent of all deaths from bronchitis and emphysema can be attributed to smoking.

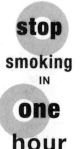

stop
smoking
IN
one
hour

Smoking causes:

 damage to and loss of efficiency in the lungs

 recurrent infections in the airways

 chronic bronchitis, emphysema and other lung diseases

In 1972, 52 per cent of men and 41 per cent of women smoked cigarettes – nearly half the adult population of the UK. Now just over one-quarter smoke, but the decline in recent years has been heavily concentrated in older age groups and more established smokers. Many young people are becoming smokers.

Smoking numbers are highest among those aged 20–24: 36 per cent of women and 43 per cent of men in this age group smoke. Smoking levels remain higher than the national average among both men and women until they reach the age of 50–59.

The majority of people who become smokers do so in adolescence rather than adulthood.

Of the 12 million smokers in the UK (50 million in the US), more than two-thirds say they would like to become non-smokers.

According to UK Government figures, 1,000 people in the UK become non-smokers every day, however more than double that amount attempt to become non-smokers and fail.

I am confident that if I conducted a survey around the world and asked every smoker, 'If you could become a non-smoker and it was easy, would you do it?' The majority would say, 'Yes, absolutely.'

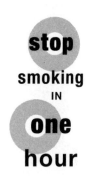

Some 480,000
Americans die prematurely
of smoking-related
diseases each year.

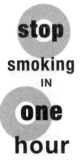

stop
smoking
IN
one
hour

More and more public places are becoming 'smoke-free' zones. Companies are introducing 'no-smoking' policies.

Smoking kills around six times more people in the UK than all the following causes put together (based on 1996 figures):

 road traffic accidents (3,647)

 murder and manslaughter (448)

 suicide (4,175)

 poisoning and overdoses (1,071)

 HIV infection (577)

 all other accidents (9,974)

Tobacco use kills more people in the US every year than alcohol, cocaine, crack, heroin, road traffic accidents, homicides, ETS and HIV combined.

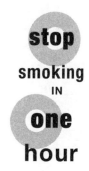

stop
smoking
IN
one
hour

How Smoking Affects Teenagers

Most children hate smoking and will make gestures or comments to that effect when in the company of adults who are smoking. However, an alarming number of these go on to become smokers themselves.

When teenagers become smokers they immediately put themselves at risk of:

 life-long dependency on tobacco

 the likelihood of facing minor illnesses in the early years

 the likelihood of suffering from serious diseases later in life

 being less fit and generally suffering poorer health.

Polls show that the public overestimates the number of people who smoke, and underestimates the dangers of smoking. It is especially easy for young people to underestimate how dangerous smoking is.

A common myth among young smokers is that death and smoking-related diseases do not happen to them, only to their parents and grandparents.

About 450 children in the UK – and 3,000 in the US – start smoking every day.

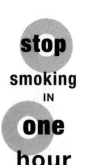

stop smoking IN one hour

Women who smoke and take the contraceptive pill have 10 times the risk of suffering a heart attack, stroke or other cardiovascular disease compared with those who take the contraceptive pill but are non-smokers.

Smoking has also been linked with an increased likelihood of menstrual problems (although not with PMT).

Smoking leads to an earlier menopause: on average women smokers go through the menopause up to 2 years earlier than non-smokers.

Women who smoke are at a greater risk of developing osteoporosis (loss of bony tissue, resulting in brittle bones that are liable to fracture). Smoking reduces bone density; a woman who smokes 20 cigarettes a day throughout adulthood is left with a 5–10 per cent reduction in bone density at the onset of menopause. This would be sufficient to increase the risk of fracture.

Risks of Smoking During Pregnancy

Smoking during pregnancy leads to an increased risk of:

 spontaneous abortion (miscarriage) and other problems during pregnancy

 bleeding during pregnancy causing unnecessary worry

 low birthweight babies

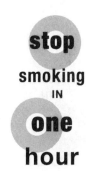

**Tobacco
is the only legally
available consumer
product which kills people
when it is used entirely
as intended.**

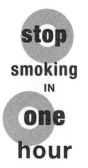

stop
smoking
IN
one
hour

Smoking has been associated with:

 increased sperm abnormalities

 impotence

The Chemicals in Tobacco Smoke

Tobacco smoke reportedly contains over 600 chemicals, present either as gases or as tiny particles.[20] Of these 600 chemicals, some are toxic, some are mutagenic (causing changes to your body's cells), at least 43 are known carcinogens (cancer-causing in humans), and many affect both your physical and mental function (memory, etc.).

Nicotine

One of the most addictive substances known to man, nicotine is a powerful and fast-acting poison. It stimulates the central nervous system, increasing the heart rate, making the heart work harder and raising the blood pressure. Nicotine also makes the blood sticky, which results in clots forming more easily, leading to thrombosis.

In large quantities nicotine is extremely poisonous. When a smoker inhales tobacco smoke, nicotine is absorbed into the brain and bloodstream and the effects are felt in about seven seconds.

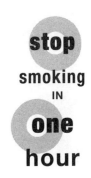

Tar is deposited in the lungs and respiratory system and gradually absorbed when you inhale on a lighted cigarette. Once inhaled, the smoke condenses and about 70 per cent of the tar in the smoke is deposited in the smoker's lungs.

Many of the substances in tar are known to cause cancer and to damage the lungs by narrowing the bronchioles and the ciliostasis (small hairs which help to protect the lungs from infection).

Tar is a mixture of many different chemicals, including:

 Formaldehyde – used to preserve dead bodies and known to cause cancer

 Arsenic – a well-known poison, fatal when used in large quantities

 Cyanide – another well-known poison, fatal when used in large quantities

 Benzene – used as a solvent in fuel and in chemical manufacture, a known carcinogen and associated with leukaemia

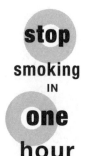

Carbon Monoxide (CO)

Carbon monoxide is a poisonous gas and found in relatively high concentration in cigarette smoke – it is the same gas that is emitted from car exhausts. Carbon monoxide impairs the circulation of oxygen in the blood by combining readily with haemoglobin (the substance which carries oxygen in the blood) more easily than oxygen does.

The oxygen levels in a smoker's blood may be reduced by 15 per cent due to carbon monoxide levels in the body, which inevitably cuts down the efficiency of a smoker's breathing.

By 2006 there will be a complete ban on all tobacco advertising and sponsorship throughout the EU.

When you consider that oxygen is essential for body tissues and cells to function efficiently, in particular to breathe more easily, then you will understand that if the supply of oxygen is reduced for long periods, breathing difficulties will develop, as will problems with growth, repair and the absorption of essential nutrients.

Carbon monoxide is therefore particularly harmful during pregnancy as it reduces the amount of essential oxygen carried to the foetus.

Tobacco Advertising

It is estimated that the tobacco industry currently spends over £100 million every year on advertising and promoting tobacco. This will be phased out as the 1998 European Union Tobacco Advertising Directive comes into full force.

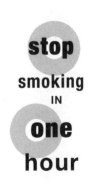

stop smoking
IN
one hour

how your
smoking
habit
controls
you

Over the years, some of my clients have told me that smoking makes them feel confident and relaxed. Are you one of those smokers with an illusion that you enjoy virtually every cigarette/cigar/pipe-full of tobacco you have?

Perhaps the reverse is true for you, in that you detest the smell, the taste and everything that accompanies smoking?

How many times have you suffered anxiety at the prospect of running out of cigarettes late at night? It is of course the anticipation of the consequences of having no cigarettes that causes the anxiety.

You sleep, on average, eight hours a night. I have never come across anyone who wakes up during the night for a cigarette. If you do smoke during the night, it is more likely that you have woken up for

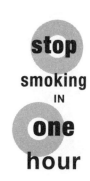

stop
smoking
IN
one
hour

There is absolutely
nothing to fear,
and you will enjoy life
even more without
smoking tobacco.

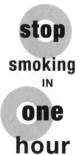

stop
smoking
IN
one
hour

some other reason and decide to have a cigarette while you are up, especially if you cannot get back to sleep.

Consider a smoker in a meeting with a non-smoker. Providing that the meeting finishes on schedule there are no problems. However, if the meeting goes on and on with no end in sight, the smoker invariably becomes disadvantaged because agitation sets in and concentration is affected as the smoker's mind inevitably drifts to thoughts of, 'When can I have a cigarette?'

Most smokers can quite happily abstain from smoking in the following situations:

 in cars

 in the company of non-smokers

 on a long-haul flight

 at the theatre or movies

 in hospital, whether for a short stay or long stay

Of course there are always the exceptions, where someone will actually leave the theatre to have a smoke, go to the smoking room in a hospital, or risk getting caught smoking in the toilet on a non-smoking long-haul flight.

Some clients who have attended my clinics are quite ashamed that they have been deceiving their partners for many months into believing that they are non-smokers. They've gone for lengthy periods

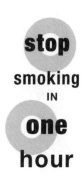

stop

smoking

IN

one

hour

without smoking during the evenings and at weekends without any real hardship, and gone to great lengths to conceal their smoking habit.

I have even known clients who have enjoyed a two-week break without smoking because their partner either is not aware of their continued habit or vehemently opposes it. At the first opportunity on their return to work they will eagerly have a cigarette as if they have been deprived, and probably wonder how they had managed for so long without smoking.

When you have attempted to become a non-smoker or have even thought about quitting during your smoking 'career', it is usually with dread because the thoughts that enter into your mind are dreadful memories of the withdrawal symptoms that you most probably have experienced in the past. It is common knowledge that most smokers believe that they will suffer withdrawal symptoms, and if you *expect* something to happen, it will. The mind is very powerful. Yet for this very same reason, using the power of your mind you can become a non-smoker easily and instantly.

Let us assume you enjoy a smoke and you also enjoy other things too, such as alcohol and/or chocolate. Then, say, for whatever reason you decide to embark on a self-improvement programme by eating more healthily, reducing your alcohol intake and attempting to become a non-smoker. Many of my clients over the years have been puzzled about why they can master other habits but not tobacco. The answer lies in *perception*.

We are bombarded with information from all sources about how addictive tobacco is and how difficult it is to become a non-smoker, so we assume that it must be virtually impossible to kick the habit.

You do not control your smoking habit. It controls you.

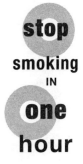

But it is all in the mind … it is not difficult to become a non-smoker and it is not to be feared but to be welcomed. It is a time of celebration. Yes, celebration, because you are rejoicing in your ability to be instrumental in enjoying a healthier and fitter life and in extending your life.

Most smokers are disappointed with themselves and feel inadequate, weak willed, frustrated and often ashamed when they fail yet again to become a non-smoker. Many have attempted several times to quit during their smoking 'career'. It does seem to the smoker that relief is felt the moment they light up, and therefore an association is made between cigarettes and pleasure. This association becomes embedded in the mind. However, I will reiterate, this is an illusion.

Every time a smoker experiences pain in the chest, shortness of breath, the death of a family member or friend from a smoking-related disease, or 'National No Smoking Day'/'American Smoke-Out Day' – to name but a few examples – guilt or reality hits and thoughts turn to the idea of becoming a non-smoker.

How Smoking Affects Your Emotions

Nicotine is one of the fastest-acting drugs known to man. When a smoker inhales tobacco smoke, the nicotine is absorbed into the bloodstream and the effects are felt almost immediately. Conversely, levels of nicotine drop quickly to about one-quarter within one hour after finishing a cigarette, hence most smokers will think they need a cigarette every hour (on average).

stop
smoking
IN
one
hour

I've heard many times of a relative who has smoked 40 cigarettes a day for over 50 years and lived to be 80. Indeed, my own grandfather was in that category and rarely had a day's illness in his life. He would never have entertained the idea of becoming a non-smoker.

Do not be fooled into thinking that you'll get away with this too. Such people are the exception.

When an octogenarian visits my clinic, the main reason he or she gives for wanting to become a non-smoker is, 'Every month is a bonus and if I can extend my life then it is worth the effort.' Their determination and willingness to try hypnosis is always uplifting.

Excuses, Excuses

When you are a smoker it is extremely easy to find excuses for why you smoke and to believe that it is the answer to all your problems. When you are unable to concentrate, you are convinced that you will be able to concentrate when you light up a cigarette.

When someone irritates you, you are convinced that you will feel more relaxed when you light up a cigarette. When first you become a non-smoker, everything that goes wrong is blamed on the fact that you are not smoking. Your partner urges you to buy some cigarettes because you are irritable and no longer a pleasure to be with. Do any of these scenarios sound familiar?

The fact is, smoking never made anyone perfect. Even smokers get irritable, have trouble concentrating and are not always a pleasure to be with. You can't pin these or any other problems on the fact that you are a non-smoker. You have not changed, your personal circumstances have probably not changed, you will still get cross, but it is very easy to blame these emotions on being a non-smoker because we are constantly bombarded with information about how smoking relaxes you and releases stress. We tell ourselves that it does seem to be a consensus of opinion so it must be right!

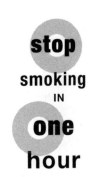

Smokers are constantly on a roller-coaster with their emotions, agitated when they cannot get a cigarette if they want one and at the same time agitated when they smoke. This is due, to a large extent, by the very nature of the habit and the frustration caused by being controlled by an outside force, something that feels beyond your control.

Yet most smokers continue to find excuses to put off the day they'll become non-smokers. Smokers also act under the illusion that the innumerable statistics written about the dangers of smoking are overstated. Reading the statistics contained in this book makes for alarming reading. You might think that these statistics alone are enough to frighten anyone into either becoming a non-smoker or never to start smoking in the first place.

Well, smokers do not want to know about the statistics until they decide to become non-smokers. If they really *believed* that cigarettes were going to kill them, give them cancer or be instrumental in the amputation of a leg, would they smoke another cigarette?

How Smoking Affects the Skin

While smoking has a detrimental effect on the internal organs, particularly the heart and lungs, it also has a noticeable ageing effect on the skin, in particular the skin colour and the likelihood of early wrinkles.

stop smoking IN one hour

Environmental Tobacco Smoke (ETS) has a drying effect on the skin's surface, and smoking restricts blood vessels, reducing the amount of blood flowing to the skin. This depletes the skin of oxygen and essential nutrients. Research suggests that smoking may reduce the body's store of vitamin A, which provides protection against some skin-damaging agents produced by smoking.

Smoking affects healing of the skin and, noticeably, wounds in smokers (this includes surgical incisions) take longer to heal.

Cigars to Have Health Warnings

ASH in the US have filed a petition asking the Federal Trade Commission (FTC) to require 'cigarette-like' health warnings on cigars. In view of new evidence that cigar smoking is as dangerous as cigarette smoking – and that cigar smoking is becoming increasingly popular among young people – victory was achieved.

The risks of smoking pipes and cigars, compared to cigarettes, are difficult to assess – it depends on whether the smoker inhales the smoke or not. Smokers who inhale pipe and cigar smoke are just as much at risk of developing lung cancer as cigarette smokers. However, all cigar and pipe smokers have a higher risk of developing cancers of the lip, mouth and throat than cigarette smokers.

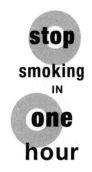

why
sm•ke?

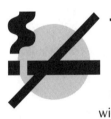

That First Cigarette

Do you remember your first cigarette or why you started to smoke in the first place? Most smokers will give similar answers to these two questions. For most it is something they did because their family or friends did it. Most smokers can remember that they felt dreadful after their first puff, which probably left them feeling faint and nauseated. You may have been one of these, but you probably said to yourself, 'I will persevere. I will enjoy them. All my friends enjoy them so I will too.'

You may have felt that you had joined the 'gang' when you had completed the initiation ceremony of having your first cigarette. The transition for you into the mysterious adult world (as many smokers begin during their teens) is helped along by the impression that smoking made you look sophisticated and of course 'grown up', and therefore made you feel more confident. Does this sound familiar?

stop
smoking
IN
one
hour

Then – perhaps after many years of smoking – something changes within you, or your circumstances change, and this makes you spend several more years trying to extricate yourself from the habit.

Perhaps you have become a parent and feel guilty about putting your child's health at risk, or maybe you are planning to start a family and preparing your body for that event. Maybe it is simply the tremendous amount of publicity regarding health risks associated with smoking that has made you realize you cannot ignore the dangers any longer. Whatever your reasons for becoming a non-smoker, it is an excellent decision, one that you will not regret and one that will lengthen your life.

The majority of my clients have had a smoking 'career' in that they have made several attempts at becoming non-smokers and succumbed to the temptation of that one cigarette, spurred on by some kind of crisis, an inability to concentrate or a party or setting where everyone else seems to be smoking.

Even if you have never attempted to become a non-smoker, you may have experienced irritability and panicky feelings when you discover that you've run out of cigarettes and the shops are closed. You may also recall fellow-smokers discussing their withdrawal symptoms.

Becoming a non-smoker is different for everyone. Different people suffer varying degrees of anxiety, but absolutely no one enjoys it. It is natural to be apprehensive about the unknown, but you need not fear becoming a non-smoker with this method.

I do understand and sympathize totally. It's one of the reasons that I set myself the task of helping as many people as I could to become non-smokers. However, I do have another reason, a personal one.

stop
smoking
IN
one
hour

In 1977 I lost my very dear mother to a smoking-related disease when she was 54 years of age. I later discovered that my mother had been told by her doctor that she must stop smoking or it would prove fatal. She, like many others, thought that her doctor's words were just shock tactics. Like many others, she believed on some level that it would never happen to her. I was absolutely devastated at my mother's death and had no idea that smoking cigarettes was so deadly (back then we certainly did not have the same publicity regarding the dangers of smoking that we have now).

When I qualified as a hypnotherapist, I spent many years hoping and actively trying to persuade my husband and my twin sister to become non-smokers, even though I knew they had to *want* to do it for themselves. Incidentally, much to my delight, they both asked for my help 10 years ago, and happily have never touched the dreadful tobacco since.

From my records covering over 14 years, the majority of my clients have smoked a minimum of 40 cigarettes a day, which costs over £50 per week in the UK (and runs to about $45 in the US); this equates to a staggering £2,920 ($2,560) a year at current prices. Some of my clients (albeit very few, I'm pleased to say) have smoked 80—100 cigarettes a day, which equates to over £6,000 ($5,800) a year and *very bad health*.

Some doctors refuse to treat patients who smoke; indeed, you may have been on the receiving end of this kind of policy. I have certainly treated clients who are anxious to become non-smokers because they have been diagnosed as having arteriosclerosis (hardening of the arteries) and have been told that unless they become non-smokers they will most probably lose a leg.

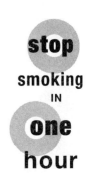

stop smoking IN one hour

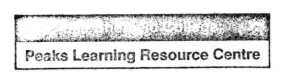

These particular clients usually have a sense of sadness and frustration that they have to enlist outside help to become non-smokers, as they feel that the threat of losing a leg should be incentive enough. Yet so insidious is the habit, that even people who know they have a life-threatening illness, which is exacerbated by the smoking habit, find becoming a non-smoker virtually impossible. For whatever reason, some of my clients, before they heard about my treatment methods, were under the impression that becoming a non-smoker was an insurmountable hurdle and had given up trying.

I have helped many thousands of smokers over the years to become non-smokers, and the obvious delight in their voices when they tell me that they are non-smokers is sometimes overwhelmingly moving. It is also overwhelming whenever anyone informs me that they have not managed to succeed. Fortunately these are few and far between.

Some of the most common comments I hear in my clinic:

☞ 'If my sister/friend/colleague, etc. can stop smoking, I know I can, too.'

☞ 'I can't really believe that I will ever be without cigarettes, but it would be wonderful. It is very exciting.'

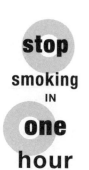

stop
smoking
IN
one
hour

☞ 'The thought of never having a cigarette again terrifies me; I wonder how I will cope in a crisis without them?'

☞ 'My friend came to see you for this treatment and she said it was very easy, she hasn't put weight on either, but I will probably be one of the 10 per cent who either struggles or doesn't manage to become a non-smoker. It seems too good to be true.'

☞ 'I have been counting every day since I made my appointment. I feel it's extraordinary that I can walk out of here and not smoke again. It would be wonderful. I would feel free. I always felt it was just a matter of time before I stopped smoking.'

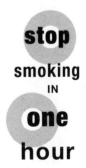

stop smoking IN **one** hour

success stories

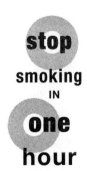

One woman who came to me for help with stopping smoking had been told at the age of 30 that if she didn't stop smoking she would lose a leg before she was 40, because of an inherited narrowing of the arteries. Her mother had lost a leg at the age of 40, as had her maternal grandmother, at the age of 42. This woman and mother of four young children came to see me when she was 36, after spending years asking herself repeatedly, 'why can't I stop smoking?' Happily this woman is now a non-smoker and all problems with her legs have improved.

Another woman who phoned me one day to enquire about my treatment often comes into my thoughts. She was due to go away on holiday and said that she would wait until she came back, as she was sharing a villa with nine others and, if past holidays were anything to go by, they would all be smoking heavily (duty-free cigarettes) during the holiday and she thought it would be difficult to resist having a cigarette.

stop smoking IN **one hour**

I told her that it was entirely up to her, but assured her that it would make no difference whether she had the treatment before going on holiday or on her return: providing she really wanted to become a non-smoker for *herself*, then she should succeed and would not be affected by others' smoking. She decided to see me before her holiday, and was so amazed that she simply did not want a cigarette at all, that on her return she brought some of her friends and several members of her family along – including her 75-year-old uncle!

A young woman named Claire came to see me several years ago. When her mother Sandra phoned her to congratulate her on being a non-smoker, Claire asserted that, much to her disappointment, the treatment hadn't worked, saying 'I wasn't even hypnotized.' Yet the next day, over lunch, their conversation went something like this:

Sandra: **What a great shame about the hypnosis. I had really pinned my hopes on that working.**

Claire: **Oh, actually, now that you mention it, I've forgotten to have a cigarette today.**

Sandra: **What do you mean you've forgotten to have a cigarette? How can you forget?**

Claire: **Well, I have.**

Sandra: **Did you have a cigarette last night?**

Claire: **No, but I didn't want one.**

Sandra: **Well, if you didn't have a cigarette last night and you have 'forgotten' to have one today, then it seems to me the hypnosis worked after all!**

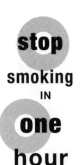

stop smoking IN **one** hour

Claire: It can't have, Mum, I wasn't even hypnotized.

Sandra: Claire, you have never lasted more than a few hours without a cigarette before. I'd say it must have worked!

Claire remains a non-smoker.

A gentleman named Tom came to see me recently and said, 'I have to say it was incredibly easy and I was rather worried initially that it would wear off. I attended a function some 24 hours later and others were smoking. I found it truly amazing that I didn't want a cigarette. I don't even notice when others are smoking any more.'

I have seen many clients over the years who have been most upset by the comments made by their partners, to the effect that they 'smell terrible' and that kissing them 'is most unpleasant'. I have also known of clients whose partners threaten to end the relationship unless they become non-smokers (usually this only happens with fairly new relationships). Often this is due to the smoker having deceived the partner by insisting that they have given up, only to then get 'caught out'.

Finally, I have treated many employees from a particular chain of restaurants. Amazingly, one of the managers was so delighted to become a non-smoker after 30 years of trying other methods, he appears to have taken on a personal mission to refer every smoking customer, friend, family member and colleague to visit my clinic.

I discovered recently that a customer from his restaurant (who had been referred to me by this particular manager) was so delighted to become a non-smoker that she presented him with armfuls of presents: champagne, flowers and chocolates. She told him, 'You have given me the best present ever in my life and I want to say a big thank you.'

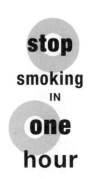

stop smoking IN **one hour**

Here, to help you with your resolve, is a sample of letters I've received from clients (printed with their permission).

How can I thank you for my freedom after all these years? You have shown that it can be done, even after 50 years of smoking. I am now a non-smoker with grateful thanks.

I have tried every method to stop smoking without success, but this time it definitely feels different and I know that I shall never smoke again. Thank you for my freedom, I feel new again.

I have not had a cigarette for one year now, after only one session with you. After smoking 100 cigarettes a day, this is quite an achievement. I could not have done it without your help. Thank you very much and may you continue in your wonderful work.

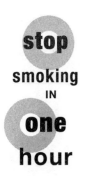

stop smoking IN **one** hour

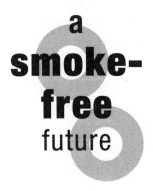

a smoke-free future

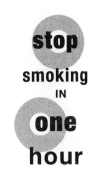

stop smoking IN one hour

A Brief History of Cigarette Smoking and Lung Cancer

Lung cancer was very rare before the introduction of cigarettes. Researchers looking through the pre-1900 medical literature have found references to only 100 cases of lung cancer.[21]

In the 19th century, tobacco was smoked by the gentry in the form of cigars. The general workforce would make the sweepings off the floor into cigars and smoke them.

Since there is a time-lag of approximately 20 years between the time a person starts smoking and the development of lung cancer, the damage caused by tobacco was not immediately apparent. However, in the 1930s, a dramatic increase in lung cancer in men helped the medical establishment make the connection between smoking and the disease. By the 1970s lung cancer had moved from being one of the rarest forms of the disease to being the number one cancer killer in the Western world.

Women rarely smoked in the early 20th century, and thus the incidence of lung cancer in women was extremely rare. An intensive advertising campaign begun in the 1930s and portraying elegant women smoking cigarettes in fine cigarette holders changed all this. Smoking came to be associated with 'sophistication'. Nevertheless, by the early 1970s lung cancer in women was still unusual – but by 1985, it was the number one cause of cancer deaths in women.

ASH

I would like to take this opportunity to provide you with some information about ASH (Action on Smoking and Health) – the UK and US organizations which we all have to thank for their involvement and instrumental role in effecting many changes made towards ensuring we live in a cleaner and healthier environment.

ASH (UK) provides information on all aspects of tobacco issues and works to advance policies and measures that will help to prevent the addiction, disease and unnecessary premature death caused by smoking.

They are often accused of being anti-smoking, but they are not. They work tirelessly to secure public, media, parliamentary and local and national government support for a comprehensive programme to tackle the epidemic of tobacco-related disease. Their work and aims include:

stop
smoking
IN
one
hour

working to see a ban on all forms of tobacco advertising, sponsorship and promotion

 a major communications programme aimed at encouraging smokers to become non-smokers and non-smokers never to start smoking

 increasing the number of smoke-free public places

 improving health warnings

 the enforcement of appropriate restrictions on retailers

 the regulation of tobacco as a dangerous drug with controls over the contents of cigarettes and smoke

ASH works by highlighting the scale of the problem to decision makers, the public and the media, to create a greater understanding. They are active in lobbying to ensure that tobacco control measures are introduced and to secure political support to make things happen.

ASH (US) is the largest and oldest anti-smoking organization in the US. Founded by John F Banzhaf in 1969, it has played a major role in the non-smokers' rights movement. Its actions have helped to prohibit cigarette commercials, ban smoking on planes, buses and in many public places, and lower insurance premiums for non-smokers. ASH (US) is supported entirely by private citizens concerned about smoking and the rights of non-smokers.

An invaluable and succinct statement from ASH (UK) runs as follows:

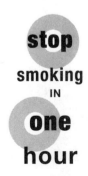

☞ We do not advocate banning smoking or making it illegal. However, the impact of tobacco smoke on other people (workers in smoky areas, partners at home, and the children of smokers) means there is a clash between the freedom to smoke and the freedom from smoke. In our view, the right to clean air takes precedence over the right to fill a common space with a substance that causes cancer, heart disease and respiratory illness. This means that there must be restrictions on where people can smoke.

As I have been working for the past 14 years in my capacity as a hypnotherapist, helping many thousands of clients to become non-smokers, I know that cynics would suggest that governments will never do anything to help smokers give up the habit, as this would jeopardize the tobacco revenue. This is simply not true.

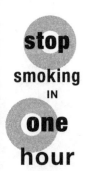

APPENDIX

smoking kills –

a uk government

white paper ON

tobacco

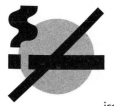

I have extracted certain facts from the UK government's 'White Paper on Tobacco' published in December 1998 (the first ever in the UK on smoking), to give you an insight into some of the issues the government are addressing. The paper begins with a powerful statement from Prime Minister Tony Blair, demonstrating his great concern for the welfare of the British people.

You may find that some of the Government statistics duplicate the statistics provided by ASH, but this is because ASH and the Government work closely and the source of information is sometimes the same.

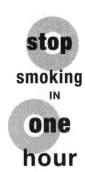

Smoking kills. In Britain today, more than 120,000 people are going to die over the next year from illnesses directly related to smoking. For the European Union as a whole, the number of deaths from tobacco is

stop smoking IN **one hour**

**Smoking
kills more than
13 people an hour.**

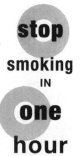

estimated at well over 500,000 a year. In the US this figure stands at 480,000 deaths every year. This trend will only continue unless we all do something.

These statistics are indeed difficult to grasp and, all too often, too easy to dismiss in that 'it will not happen to me' syndrome. They are powerful statistics and are a reminder and a testimony to individual and family suffering which need not and should not happen.

This appalling waste of people's lives is extremely frustrating, as it is *preventable*. We all have a choice, so when anyone chooses to become a non-smoker, they have chosen prolonged life over an earlier death.

We all have a responsibility to help each other, both smokers and non-smokers have rights and responsibilities – to themselves, to each other, to their families, and to the wider community. The Government is determined to meet its responsibilities. The White Paper on tobacco is a key part in ensuring that the Government keeps its promise, and is a significant step towards achieving the goal of improving public health for all the people of Britain.

Smoking kills, there is no getting away from this crucial fact. This has been known for years, hence why many adults have become non-smokers. But sadly the number of children who smoke is increasing, with more girls than boys taking up this deadly habit.

Smoking is the principal avoidable cause of premature deaths in the UK. Smoking harms babies in the womb and causes numerous diseases, often debilitating, sometimes fatal. Passive smoking carries the same dangers albeit to a lesser extent and often these dangers are overlooked.

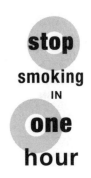

stop smoking IN **one hour**

The Government is determined to help smokers to become non-smokers and to raise awareness among children and young people to avoid becoming smokers in the first instance. These objectives can only be achieved by a concerted campaign to reduce smoking, and a major part of the effort will be targeted on children – essential when you consider that the vast majority of smokers start as teenagers and many will go on to be regular smokers for the rest of their lives.

The Government is taking positive action. A European-wide ban on tobacco advertising and sponsorship is being introduced. This will be backed up by a powerful £50 million publicity campaign.

Smoking is the single greatest cause of preventable illness and premature death in the UK. We simply cannot afford to ignore the dangers any longer.

Cancer and heart disease are the two most common fatal diseases. Smoking is a major cause of cancer and heart disease.

The Government's new targets will reinforce their key goals for public health improvement. They include improving the health of the nation as a whole, by increasing the length of people's lives and the number of years people spend free from illness. It cannot be done unless we tackle smoking.

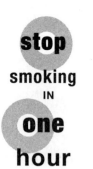

According to World Health Organization statistics, smokers in the UK smoke about 25 per cent more than the EU average, though actual smoking rates in the UK are roughly at the average for the EU as a whole.

Regular smokers who die of a smoking-related disease lose on average 16 years from their life expectancy compared to non-smokers.

 For every 1,000 smokers, 500 will die of the habit if they continue to smoke for most of their lives.

 For every 1,000 20-year-old smokers, it is estimated that while one will be murdered and six will die in motor accidents, 250 will die in middle age from smoking, and 250 will die in older age from smoking.

 Smoking causes one out of every seven deaths from heart disease, and 40,300 deaths a year in the UK from all circulatory diseases.

 Smoking is also linked to many other serious conditions including asthma and brittle bone disease (osteoporosis).

 The UK's National Health Service (NHS) spends up to £1.7 billion every year in terms of doctors' time, prescriptions, treatment and operations to combat illnesses caused by smoking.

 Passive smoking also kills. While most non-smokers are not exposed to levels of passive smoke sufficient for them to incur significant extra risk, many thousands are, such as those living with smokers or working in particularly smoky atmospheres for long periods of time. Non-smokers and smokers need to be made aware of the risks.

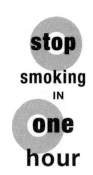

stop
smoking
IN
one
hour

Tobacco use kills around 120,000 people in the UK every year.

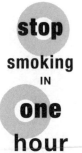

stop
smoking
IN
one
hour

Several hundred people a year in the UK are estimated to die from lung cancer brought about by passive smoking. Passive smoking almost certainly contributes to deaths from heart disease – an even bigger killer than lung cancer.

 Passive smoking, even in low levels, can cause illness. Asthma sufferers are more prone to attacks in smoky atmospheres.

 Children, more vulnerable than adults and often with little choice over their exposure to tobacco smoke, are at particular risk.

Government Action

The Government recognizes that:

Tobacco is a uniquely dangerous product. If introduced today, it would not stand the remotest chance of being legal. But smoking is not against the law.

Currently, well over a quarter of the adult population of Britain smoke. The Government fully recognizes their right to choose and freedom to smoke. The Government will not infringe upon that right in any of their proposals, but the Government recognizes that it also has a responsibility to those who choose not to smoke.

The Government has a clear responsibility to protect children from tobacco.

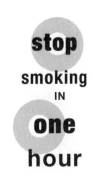

stop smoking IN one hour

The Government's proposals in the White Paper set out the major steps they intend to take. To support this new programme of action, more than £100 million will be spent over the next three years. They recognize the scale of the challenge we all face to reduce smoking and to improve the overall health of everyone, smokers and non-smokers alike.

In partnership with others and in particular ASH (Action on Health and Smoking), they are determined to meet that challenge.

I shall endeavour to play my part in this most crucial quest to make our world a healthier and safer place to live. I want to play a crucial role in ensuring an awareness of the dangers of smoking, (whether first-hand smoking or passive smoking). I shall do this through my book and CD, through lectures worldwide, interviews worldwide and any other medium to get this message across loud and clear.

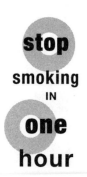

The Government have set three challenging and crucial targets for the year 2010:

(1) children smoking

(2) adults smoking

(3) smoking during pregnancy.

Children Smoking

The Government's immediate aim is to stop the increase in children smoking, and ultimately for child smokers to become non-smokers. This is seen as the most challenging area, as most smokers begin in the teenage years. It is also essential if the downward trend in adult smoking levels is to continue in the future, and if continued decline in cancer and heart disease deaths in generations to come is to be secured.

If the Government succeeds in its target to reduce smoking among children from 13 to 9 per cent or less by the year 2010 (with a fall to 11 per cent by the year 2005), this will mean approximately 110,000 fewer children smoking in England by the year 2010.

NOTE
This target is for improvements measured against a base line of 13 per cent of 11- to 15-year-olds (as of 1996) who smoke at least one cigarette a week.

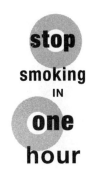

Adults Smoking

The aim here is to maintain the downward trend in smoking among the adult population.

Smoking During Pregnancy

This is a special issue because the health of the foetus is at great risk both during pregnancy and after the birth, from breathing parental smoke during childhood. Smoking undoubtedly harms the unborn child and leads to lower birthweight. New evidence also shows that women who smoke during pregnancy pass harmful carcinogens on to their baby.

Some 24 per cent of women smoke during pregnancy, and only 33 per cent of women smokers give up during pregnancy.

Children of smoking parents are more likely to suffer illness or even cot death. They are also much more likely to take up smoking themselves.

If the Government succeeds in the target to improve the health of expectant mothers and to reduce the percentage of women who smoke during pregnancy from 23 to 15 per cent by the year 2010 (with a fall to 18 per cent by the year 2005), this will mean approximately 55,000 fewer women in England smoking during pregnancy.

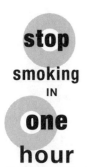

We are all becoming increasingly aware and insisting on a healthy environment and clean air, for both our work and social life. Public attitudes have certainly changed over the last two decades and businesses that fail to recognize this will increasingly find customers voting with their feet. The vast majority of people agree that smoking should be restricted in public places. Some 42 per cent consider the availability of a non-smoking area when choosing a restaurant.

At present, non-smokers are exposed to the health risks, discomfort and irritation of tobacco smoke, while smokers are often forced to smoke on the street. This naturally leads to friction and aggravation between the two camps.

Passive Smoking

The health risks are clear. Passive smoking does carry risks, albeit to a lesser extent, but hundreds die every year in the UK as a result of high levels of exposure to passive smoke.

A non-smoker living or working in an excessively smoky environment over a prolonged period is 20–30 per cent more likely to get cancer than a non-smoker who does not live or work in this type of environment.

Conclusion

The UK Government, using evidence and international experience, have put together a balanced package of measures that will save lives.

It contains arguably the most comprehensive strategy embarked upon anywhere in the world in order to tackle smoking. It represents a huge leap forward in the Government's efforts to reduce smoking in the UK, and is a critical contribution towards reducing deaths from cancer and heart disease.

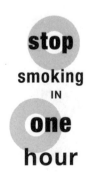

stop smoking IN one hour

Legislation is used only where required, to implement the EC Directive on the advertising and sponsorship of tobacco products.

Where possible, they have looked for partnerships:

with local government on under-age sales

with industry on a proof-of-age system

with the licensed trade on smoking in public places.

Individuals have an important role to play in looking after their own health and that of their families.

Milestones

The measures in the White Paper will quite naturally have different time scales, but the key dates are as follows:

July 2003   general tobacco sponsorship ends

2005   targets for children, adults and pregnant women

July 2006   all tobacco sponsorship ends

2010   1.5 million fewer smokers

Each measure is important for the success of the overall package.

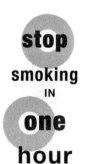

glossary

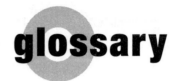

Breathing	slow and deep breathing from the diaphragm, encouraged to ensure the body enters into a state of total relaxation, which is then followed by the hypnotic state
Deepening	suggestions placed into the subconscious mind, which deepen the hypnotic state
Hypnosis	a trance-like state of intense relaxation within the body and increased awareness within the mind, similar to the state before you enter sleep, where you are neither fully asleep nor fully awake
Hypnotherapy	the treatment administered to facilitate positive changes using hypnosis

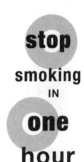

Induction	the preparation needed in order to relax the mind and body prior to the suggestions being placed, pre-hypnosis
Memory	the recall of events, relationships and situations that have been experienced
Rapid Eye Movement (REM)	the flickering of the eyelids during hypnosis (which also occurs in the dream state when you are sleeping)
Subconscious mind	the seat of all your emotions and memories
Trance	an induced state brought about by listening to the instructions of a hypnotherapist (whether in person or, as in this case, on the accompanying CD)
Visual image	mental images of positive thoughts and suggestions

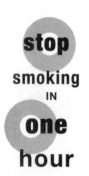

Smoking Kills

It Is Not Selective

Smoking Can Kill Anyone

Smoking Can Kill You

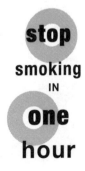

There
is absolutely
no excuse for failing
to become a **non-smoker**
with this treatment. Providing
that you want to become a non-
smoker *for yourself*,
it can be **very easy**.

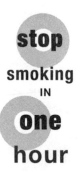

stop
smoking
IN
one
hour

references

1   American Cancer Society, 'Dangers of Smoking – Benefits of Quitting'. A.C5 1980: 8

2   Callum, C., 'The UK Smoking Epidemic: Deaths in 1995' (London HEA, 1998)

3   QUIT, Helping smokers to quit (London: QUIT, 1994; updated 1996)

4   'Respiratory health effects of passive smoking: Lung cancer and other disorders' (report of the US Environmental Protection Agency, 1993)

5   Fourth report of the Independent Scientific Committee on Smoking and Health (DHSS, 1988); 'Environmental Tobacco Smoke: Measuring exposures and assessing health effects (US National Research Council, 1986); 'Effects of passive

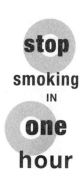

stop
smoking
IN
one
hour

smoking on health' (National Health and Medical Research Council; Australian Government Publishing, 1987)

6   Report of the Scientific Committee on Tobacco and Health (HMSO, 1998)

7   International Consultation on Environmental Tobacco Smoke (ETS) and Child Health (World Health Organization Tobacco Free Initiative; WHO/NCD/TFI/99.10, 1999)

8   'Health Effects of Exposure to Environmental Tobacco Smoke' (report of the California Environmental Protection Agency; Smoking and Tobacco Control monograph 10; National Cancer Institute, 1999)

9   Tobacco Incorporation and Prevention, 'Cigarette Smoking-related Mortality'

10 'Smoking and the Young' (a report of a working party of the Royal College of Physicians; London, 1992)

11 Hackshaw A.K., Law M., Wald N.J., 'The accumulated evidence on lung cancer and environmental tobacco smoke', *British Medical Journal* 315 (1997): 980–8

12 Boffetta, P. *et al.*, 'Multicentre case-control study of exposure to ETS and lung cancer in Europe', *Journal of the National Cancer Institute* 90 (1998): 1440–50

13 Glantz, S.A. and Parmley, W.W., 'Passive smoking and heart disease epidemiology, physiology and biochemistry',

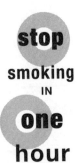

stop
smoking
IN
one
hour

Circulation 83 (1991): 1–12; '*Passive* Smoking and heart disease', *JAMA* 273.13 (1995): 1047–53

14   Law, M.R., Morris, J.K. and Wald, N.J., 'Environmental Tobacco Smoke Exposure and Ischaemic heart disease: an evaluation of the evidence', *BMJ* 315 (1997): 973–80

15   He, J. *et al.*, 'Passive smoking and the risk of coronary heart disease – a meta-analysis of epidemiology studies', *NEJM* 340 (1999): 920–6; Raitakari, O.T. *et al.*, 'Arterial endothelial dysfunction related to passive smoking is potentially reversible in healthy young adults', *Annals of Internal Medicine* 130 (1999): 578–81

16   Bonita, R. *et al.*, 'Passive smoking as well as active smoking increases the risk of acute stroke', *Tobacco Control* 8 (1999): 156–60

17   The Impact of Asthma survey (National Asthma Campaign; Allan and Hambury's Ltd, 1996)

18   Doll R., Hill A.B. 'A study of the Aetiology of Carcinoma of the Lung', *British Medical Journal* 2 (1952): 1271–86; Hammond E.C., Horn D., 'Smoking and death rates – report on 44 months of follow-up of 187,783 men', *Journal of the American Medical Association* 166 (1958): 1159–72, 1294–1308

19   Ibid.

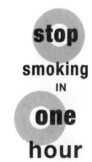

stop smoking IN one hour

20 'Reducing the health consequences of smoking: 25 years of progress' (a report of the Surgeon General, US Department of Health and Human Services, 1989)

21 Frederic W. Grannis Jr, MD, http://ourworld.compuserve.com/homepages/lungcancer

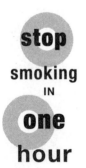

Do not leave your
future in the hands of
the tobacco companies.
They need you. You do
not need them.

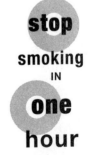

stop
smoking
IN
one
hour

From
the moment you
finish listening to
this CD you can become
a non-smoker. Thousands
of satisfied non-smokers
know it works.

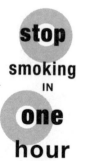

stop
smoking
IN
one
hour

The figure of 12 million smokers is based on estimates of cigarette smokers in the UK, obtained from the following sources:

Thomas M., Walker A., Bennett N., Office for National Statistics, *Living in Britain; results from the 1996 General Household Survey* (London: HMSO, 1998)

ONS Monitor Population and Health 1996, PPI 97/1 (London: Office for National Statistics, 28th August 1997)

Northern Ireland Continuous Household Survey, 1996/7 (Northern Ireland Statistics and Research Agency, 1997)

All other statistics contained in this book are from the following sources:

United States Department of Health and Human Services. 'The Health benefits of smoking cessation – a report of the Surgeon General'. US DHSS. Public Health Service, Centers for Disease Control. Center for Chronic Disease Prevention and Health Promotion. Office on Smoking and Health. DHSS Publication number (CDC) 90-8416, 1990.

ASH site: http://www.ash.org.uk/papers/basic01.html

http://ash.org/march00/03-09-00-4.html

Health Education Authority smoking site: http://www.lifesaver.co.uk

http://www.aarc.org/patient-resources/tips/quitsmok.html

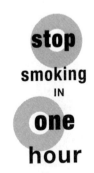
stop smoking IN one hour

useful
addresses:
choosing
a therapist

It is important that you ensure your therapist belongs to a recognized professional body.

Ideally, choose a therapist who has been recommended to you by someone you know and trust, either a member of your family or a friend. It would be preferable if the therapist has been practising for a number of years, and ensure they can deal with your particular problem.

Your doctor may be able to recommend a therapist, or you may contact one of the following organizations:

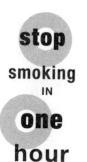

stop
smoking
IN
one
hour

The National Council for Hypnotherapy

PO Box 5779
Burton on the Wolds
Loughborough LE12 5ZF
01509 881477

The National Council for Psychotherapists

PO Box 6072
Nottingham NG6 9BW
0115 966 3062

US

The American Institute of Hypnotherapy

1805 East Garryn Avenue
Suite 100
Santa Ana, CA 92705
714-261-6400

The American Society of Clinical Hypnosis

2200 East Devon Avenue
Suite 291
Des Plaines, IL 60018
708-297-3371

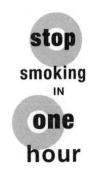